FOOD *AND* EXERCISE JOURNAL

WORK.
SWEAT.
ACHIEVE.

MY NAME

....

....

ISBN: 9781092453455

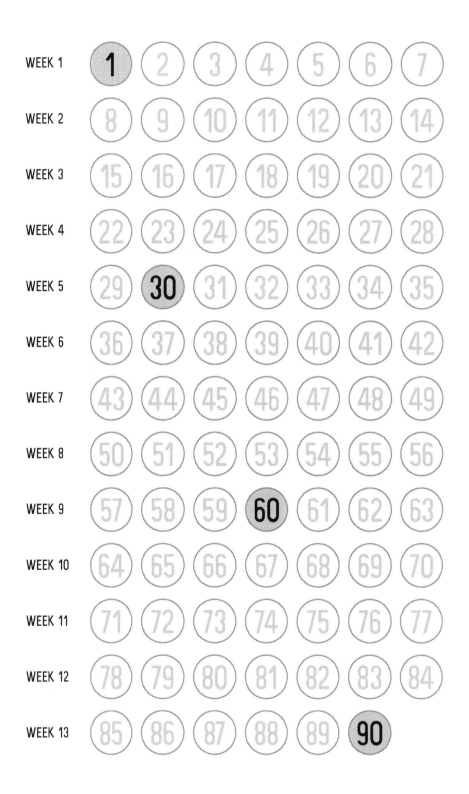

DAY 1

MY MEASUREMENTS

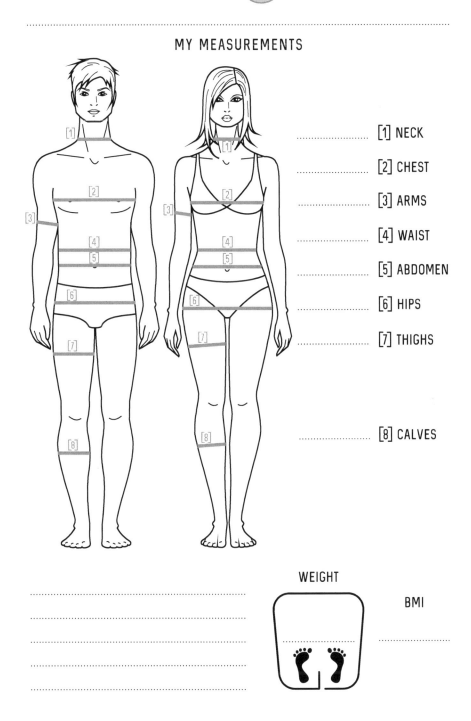

.... [1] NECK

.... [2] CHEST

.... [3] ARMS

.... [4] WAIST

.... [5] ABDOMEN

.... [6] HIPS

.... [7] THIGHS

.... [8] CALVES

WEIGHT

BMI

....

DAY (1)

MO TU WE TH FR SA SU

DATE ....

HOW I FEEL

○   ○   ○   ○

BREAKFAST
....
....
....
....
....

SNACKS
....
....
....

TOTAL CALORIES
_____

PROTEIN CONTENT   FIBER CONTENT
_____   _____

OTHER
....

LUNCH
....
....
....
....
....
....
....
....
....
....
....

DINNER
....
....
....
....
....
....
....
....
....
....
....

WEIGHT   SLEEP   WATER   PROTEIN
=========   ....

♥ EXERCISE / OTHER ACTIVITIES

EXERCISE / OTHER ACTIVITIES	SET / REPS / DISTANCE	TIME
....	....	....
....	....	....
....	....	....
....	....	....
....	....	....

NOTES
....
....

🕐 6A 7 8 9 10 11 12P 1 2 3 4 5 6 7 8 9 10+

B=BREAKFAST   L=LUNCH   D=DINNER   S=SNACKS   E=EXERCISE

HOW I FEEL

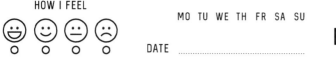

MO TU WE TH FR SA SU

DATE ....

DAY ②

BREAKFAST

....
....
....
....
....
_____ ____

SNACKS

....
....
....

TOTAL CALORIES

_____ ____

PROTEIN CONTENT FIBER CONTENT
_____ _____

OTHER

LUNCH

....
....
....
....
....
....
....
....
....
....
....
....
....
....

DINNER

....
....
....
....
....
....
....
....
....

WEIGHT   SLEEP   WATER   PROTEIN
_____ _____ ....
=============

EXERCISE / OTHER ACTIVITIES

SET / REPS / DISTANCE   TIME

....
....
....
....
....
_____ _____ _____

NOTES

....
....
....

6A 7 8 9 10 11 12P 1 2 3 4 5 6 7 8 9 10+

B=BREAKFAST L=LUNCH D=DINNER S=SNACKS E=EXERCISE

DAY (3)

MO TU WE TH FR SA SU

DATE ....

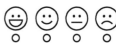

BREAKFAST
....
....
....
....
....

SNACKS
....
....
....

TOTAL CALORIES
_____

PROTEIN CONTENT   FIBER CONTENT
_____   _____

OTHER
....

LUNCH
....
....
....
....
....
....
....
....
....
....

DINNER
....
....
....
....
....
....
....
....
....
....

WEIGHT   SLEEP   WATER   PROTEIN
_____   _____   ....

 EXERCISE / OTHER ACTIVITIES   SET / REPS / DISTANCE   TIME

....
....
....
....
....

NOTES
....
....
....

 6A 7 8 9 10 11 12P 1 2 3 4 5 6 7 8 9 10+

B=BREAKFAST   L=LUNCH   D=DINNER   S=SNACKS   E=EXERCISE

HOW I FEEL

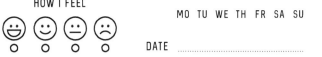

MO TU WE TH FR SA SU

DATE ....

DAY

BREAKFAST

LUNCH

DINNER

....

....

....

....

....

SNACKS

....

....

....

TOTAL CALORIES

_____

PROTEIN CONTENT FIBER CONTENT

_____ _____

OTHER

....

WEIGHT   SLEEP   WATER   PROTEIN

EXERCISE / OTHER ACTIVITIES   SET / REPS / DISTANCE   TIME

....

....

....

....

....

NOTES

....

....

6A 7 8 9 10 11 12P 1 2 3 4 5 6 7 8 9 10+

B=BREAKFAST   L=LUNCH   D=DINNER   S=SNACKS   E=EXERCISE

DAY (5)

MO TU WE TH FR SA SU

DATE ....

HOW I FEEL

BREAKFAST	LUNCH	DINNER
....	....	....
....	....	....
....	....	....
....	....	....
....	....	....
_____ __	....	....

SNACKS

....

....

....

_____ __

TOTAL CALORIES

_____

PROTEIN CONTENT   FIBER CONTENT

_____ _____

WEIGHT   SLEEP   WATER   PROTEIN

================ ....

OTHER

....

♥ EXERCISE / OTHER ACTIVITIES   SET / REPS / DISTANCE   TIME

....

....

....

....

....

_____   _____   _____

NOTES

....

....

🕐 6A 7 8 9 10 11 12P 1 2 3 4 5 6 7 8 9 10+

B=BREAKFAST   L=LUNCH   D=DINNER   S=SNACKS   E=EXERCISE

HOW I FEEL

😃 😊 😐 ☹️
○ ○ ○ ○

MO TU WE TH FR SA SU

DATE ....

DAY ⑥

BREAKFAST

....
....
....
....
....
_____ ____

SNACKS

....
....
....

TOTAL CALORIES

_____ ____

PROTEIN CONTENT FIBER CONTENT

_____ _____

LUNCH

....
....
....
....
....
....
....
....
....
....
....
....
....
....

DINNER

....
....
....
....
....

WEIGHT   SLEEP   WATER   PROTEIN

_____ ....

OTHER

....

❤️ EXERCISE / OTHER ACTIVITIES

	SET / REPS / DISTANCE	TIME
....	....	....
....	....	....
....	....	....
....	....	....
....	....	....

NOTES

....
....

🕐 6A 7 8 9 10 11 12P 1 2 3 4 5 6 7 8 9 10+

B=BREAKFAST   L=LUNCH   D=DINNER   S=SNACKS   E=EXERCISE

DAY (7)

MO TU WE TH FR SA SU

DATE ....

BREAKFAST

....
....
....
....
....
_____ ____

SNACKS

....
....
....
_____ ____

TOTAL CALORIES

_____

PROTEIN CONTENT FIBER CONTENT

_____ _____

OTHER

....

LUNCH

....
....
....
....
....
....
....
....
....
....
....

DINNER

....
....
....
....
....
....
....
....
....
....

WEIGHT   SLEEP   WATER   PROTEIN

================   ....

❤ **EXERCISE / OTHER ACTIVITIES**   SET / REPS / DISTANCE   TIME

....
....
....
....
....

NOTES

....
....

🕐 6A 7 8 9 10 11 12P 1 2 3 4 5 6 7 8 9 10+

B=BREAKFAST   L=LUNCH   D=DINNER   S=SNACKS   E=EXERCISE

HOW I FEEL

MO TU WE TH FR SA SU

DATE ....

DAY (8)

BREAKFAST

....
....
....
....
....
_____ ___ ___

SNACKS

....
....
....
_____ ____ ___

LUNCH

....
....
....
....
....
....
....
....
....
....

DINNER

....
....
....
....
....
....
....
....
....

TOTAL CALORIES

_____ ____

PROTEIN CONTENT FIBER CONTENT

_____ _____ ___

OTHER

....

WEIGHT   SLEEP   WATER   PROTEIN

❤ EXERCISE / OTHER ACTIVITIES   SET / REPS / DISTANCE   TIME

....
....
....
....
....
_____ _____ _____

NOTES

....
....
....

🕐 6A 7 8 9 10 11 12P 1 2 3 4 5 6 7 8 9 10+

B=BREAKFAST L=LUNCH D=DINNER S=SNACKS E=EXERCISE

DAY (9)

MO TU WE TH FR SA SU

DATE ....

BREAKFAST   LUNCH   DINNER

....
....
....
....
....
_____   ....

SNACKS   ....
                         ....
....
....
....
_____   ....

TOTAL CALORIES   WEIGHT   SLEEP   WATER   PROTEIN
_____

PROTEIN CONTENT FIBER CONTENT
_____ _____   _____   ....

OTHER
....

♥ EXERCISE / OTHER ACTIVITIES   SET / REPS / DISTANCE   TIME

....
....
....
....
....
_____   _____   _____

NOTES
....
....

🕐   6A 7 8 9 10 11 12P 1 2 3 4 5 6 7 8 9 10+
     B=BREAKFAST   L=LUNCH   D=DINNER   S=SNACKS   E=EXERCISE

HOW I FEEL

MO TU WE TH FR SA SU

DATE ....

DAY (10)

BREAKFAST

....
....
....
....
....

_____ ___

SNACKS

....
....
....

TOTAL CALORIES

_____ ___

PROTEIN CONTENT FIBER CONTENT

_____ _____ ____

OTHER

LUNCH

....
....
....
....
....
....
....
....
....
....
....
....

WEIGHT   SLEEP   WATER   PROTEIN

_____ .... _____

DINNER

....
....
....
....
....
....
....
....

....

EXERCISE / OTHER ACTIVITIES	SET / REPS / DISTANCE	TIME
....	....	....
....	....	....
....	....	....
....	....	....
....	....	....

NOTES

....
....

6A 7 8 9 10 11 12P 1 2 3 4 5 6 7 8 9 10+
....

B=BREAKFAST   L=LUNCH   D=DINNER   S=SNACKS   E=EXERCISE

DAY (11)

MO TU WE TH FR SA SU

DATE ....

HOW I FEEL

BREAKFAST

....
....
....
....
....

LUNCH

....
....
....
....
....
....
....
....
....

DINNER

....
....
....
....
....

SNACKS

....
....
....

TOTAL CALORIES

_____

PROTEIN CONTENT   FIBER CONTENT

_____   _____

OTHER

....

WEIGHT   SLEEP   WATER   PROTEIN

❤ EXERCISE / OTHER ACTIVITIES   SET / REPS / DISTANCE   TIME

.... | .... | ....
.... | .... | ....
.... | .... | ....
.... | .... | ....
.... | .... | ....

NOTES

....
....

🕐   6A   7   8   9   10   11   12P   1   2   3   4   5   6   7   8   9   10+

B=BREAKFAST   L=LUNCH   D=DINNER   S=SNACKS   E=EXERCISE

HOW I FEEL

☺ ☺ ☺ ☹
○ ○ ○ ○

MO TU WE TH FR SA SU

DATE ....

DAY ⑫

BREAKFAST

LUNCH

DINNER

....
....
....
....
....

SNACKS

....
....
....

TOTAL CALORIES

_____ ___

PROTEIN CONTENT FIBER CONTENT

WEIGHT

SLEEP

WATER

PROTEIN

OTHER
....

♥ EXERCISE / OTHER ACTIVITIES

SET / REPS / DISTANCE

TIME

....
....
....
....
....

NOTES
....
....

🕐 6A 7 8 9 10 11 12P 1 2 3 4 5 6 7 8 9 10+

B=BREAKFAST   L=LUNCH   D=DINNER   S=SNACKS   E=EXERCISE

DAY (13)

MO TU WE TH FR SA SU

DATE ....

HOW I FEEL

BREAKFAST

....

....

....

....

....

LUNCH

....

....

....

....

....

....

....

DINNER

....

....

....

....

....

SNACKS

....

....

....

TOTAL CALORIES

_____

PROTEIN CONTENT FIBER CONTENT

_____ _____

OTHER

....

WEIGHT   SLEEP   WATER   PROTEIN

❤ EXERCISE / OTHER ACTIVITIES

EXERCISE / OTHER ACTIVITIES	SET / REPS / DISTANCE	TIME
....	....	....
....	....	....
....	....	....
....	....	....
....	....	....

NOTES

....

....

🕐 6A 7 8 9 10 11 12P 1 2 3 4 5 6 7 8 9 10+

B=BREAKFAST L=LUNCH D=DINNER S=SNACKS E=EXERCISE

😃 😊 😐 😞
○ ○ ○ ○

MO TU WE TH FR SA SU

DATE ....

DAY (14)

BREAKFAST

....

....

....

....

....

_____ ____

SNACKS

....

....

....

_____ ____

LUNCH

....

....

....

....

....

....

....

....

....

....

....

DINNER

....

....

....

....

....

....

....

TOTAL CALORIES

_____

PROTEIN CONTENT   FIBER CONTENT

_____ _____

WEIGHT   SLEEP   WATER   PROTEIN

_____ _____ ....

OTHER

....

❤ EXERCISE / OTHER ACTIVITIES

EXERCISE / OTHER ACTIVITIES	SET / REPS / DISTANCE	TIME
....	....	....
....	....	....
....	....	....
....	....	....
....	....	....

NOTES

....

....

🕐 6A 7 8 9 10 11 12P 1 2 3 4 5 6 7 8 9 10+

B=BREAKFAST   L=LUNCH   D=DINNER   S=SNACKS   E=EXERCISE

DAY (15)

MO TU WE TH FR SA SU

DATE ....

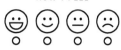

BREAKFAST

....
....
....
....
....

SNACKS

....
....
....

TOTAL CALORIES

_____

PROTEIN CONTENT   FIBER CONTENT

_____   _____

OTHER
....

LUNCH

....
....
....
....
....
....
....
....
....

DINNER

....
....
....
....
....
....
....
....

WEIGHT   SLEEP   WATER   PROTEIN

❤ EXERCISE / OTHER ACTIVITIES   SET / REPS / DISTANCE   TIME

....
....
....
....
....

NOTES

....
....

🕐 6A 7 8 9 10 11 12P 1 2 3 4 5 6 7 8 9 10+

B=BREAKFAST   L=LUNCH   D=DINNER   S=SNACKS   E=EXERCISE

HOW I FEEL

😀 😊 😐 😞
○ ○ ○ ○

MO TU WE TH FR SA SU

DATE ....

DAY (16)

BREAKFAST	LUNCH	DINNER
....		
....		
....		
....		
....		

SNACKS

....
....
....

TOTAL CALORIES

_____

PROTEIN CONTENT   FIBER CONTENT

WEIGHT   SLEEP   WATER   PROTEIN

_____   _____

OTHER
....

♡ **EXERCISE / OTHER ACTIVITIES**   SET / REPS / DISTANCE   TIME

....	....	....
....	....	....
....	....	....
....	....	....
....	....	....

NOTES
....
....

🕐 6A 7 8 9 10 11 12P 1 2 3 4 5 6 7 8 9 10+

B=BREAKFAST   L=LUNCH   D=DINNER   S=SNACKS   E=EXERCISE

DAY (17)

MO TU WE TH FR SA SU

DATE ....

BREAKFAST

....
....
....
....
....

_____

SNACKS

....
....
....

_____

TOTAL CALORIES

_____

PROTEIN CONTENT   FIBER CONTENT

_____   _____

OTHER

....

LUNCH

....
....
....
....
....
....
....
....
....
....

DINNER

....
....
....
....
....
....
....
....
....
....

WEIGHT   **SLEEP**   **WATER**   **PROTEIN**

_____   _____   ....

♥ **EXERCISE / OTHER ACTIVITIES**   SET / REPS / DISTANCE   TIME

....
....
....
....
....

_____   _____   _____

NOTES

....
....

6A 7 8 9 10 11 12P 1 2 3 4 5 6 7 8 9 10+

B=BREAKFAST   L=LUNCH   D=DINNER   S=SNACKS   E=EXERCISE

HOW I FEEL

MO TU WE TH FR SA SU

DATE ....

DAY (18)

BREAKFAST
....
....
....
....
....
_____   ___

SNACKS
....
....
....
_____   ___

TOTAL CALORIES
_____
PROTEIN CONTENT FIBER CONTENT
_____   _____

OTHER

LUNCH
....
....
....
....
....
....
....
....
....
....
....

DINNER
....
....
....
....
....
....
....
....

WEIGHT   SLEEP   WATER   PROTEIN
_____   _____   ....

EXERCISE / OTHER ACTIVITIES	SET / REPS / DISTANCE	TIME
....	....	....
....	....	....
....	....	....
....	....	....
....	....	....

NOTES
....
....

6A 7 8 9 10 11 12P 1 2 3 4 5 6 7 8 9 10+

B=BREAKFAST   L=LUNCH   D=DINNER   S=SNACKS   E=EXERCISE

DAY (19)

MO TU WE TH FR SA SU

DATE ....

BREAKFAST	LUNCH	DINNER
....	....	....
....	....	....
....	....	....
....	....	....
....	....	....

SNACKS

....

....

....

TOTAL CALORIES

_____ ___

PROTEIN CONTENT   FIBER CONTENT

WEIGHT   SLEEP   WATER   PROTEIN

_____ ___   ======

OTHER

♡ EXERCISE / OTHER ACTIVITIES   SET / REPS / DISTANCE   TIME

.... | .... | ....
.... | .... | ....
.... | .... | ....
.... | .... | ....
.... | .... | ....

NOTES

....

....

6A 7 8 9 10 11 12P 1 2 3 4 5 6 7 8 9 10+

B=BREAKFAST   L=LUNCH   D=DINNER   S=SNACKS   E=EXERCISE

HOW I FEEL

MO TU WE TH FR SA SU

DATE ....

DAY (20)

BREAKFAST

....
....
....
....
....

SNACKS

....
....
....

TOTAL CALORIES

_____

PROTEIN CONTENT   FIBER CONTENT

_____   _____

OTHER

LUNCH

....
....
....
....
....
....
....
....
....

DINNER

....
....
....
....
....
....

WEIGHT   SLEEP   WATER   PROTEIN

_____   _____   ....

EXERCISE / OTHER ACTIVITIES	SET / REPS / DISTANCE	TIME
....	....	....
....	....	....
....	....	....
....	....	....
....	....	....

NOTES

....
....

6A 7 8 9 10 11 12P 1 2 3 4 5 6 7 8 9 10+

B=BREAKFAST   L=LUNCH   D=DINNER   S=SNACKS   E=EXERCISE

DAY (21)

MO TU WE TH FR SA SU

DATE ....

BREAKFAST

....
....
....
....
....

SNACKS

....
....
....

TOTAL CALORIES

_____

PROTEIN CONTENT   FIBER CONTENT

_____   _____

OTHER

....

LUNCH

....
....
....
....
....
....
....
....
....
....
....
....
....

DINNER

....
....
....
....
....

WEIGHT   SLEEP   WATER   PROTEIN

_____   ....

❤ EXERCISE / OTHER ACTIVITIES   SET / REPS / DISTANCE   TIME

....
....
....
....
....

NOTES

....
....
....

🕐 6A 7 8 9 10 11 12P 1 2 3 4 5 6 7 8 9 10+

B=BREAKFAST   L=LUNCH   D=DINNER   S=SNACKS   E=EXERCISE

HOW I FEEL

😃 🙂 😐 ☹️
○ ○ ○ ○

MO TU WE TH FR SA SU

DATE ....

DAY (22)

BREAKFAST

....
....
....
....
....

_____ ____

SNACKS

....
....
....

_____ ____

LUNCH

....
....
....
....
....
....
....
....
....
....
....

DINNER

....
....
....
....
....
....
....
....

TOTAL CALORIES

_____

PROTEIN CONTENT FIBER CONTENT

_____ ____

WEIGHT   SLEEP   WATER   PROTEIN

_____ _____ ....

OTHER

....

♡ EXERCISE / OTHER ACTIVITIES

SET / REPS / DISTANCE   TIME

....
....
....
....
....

NOTES

....
....

🕐 | 6A | 7 | 8 | 9 | 10 | 11 | 12P | 1 | 2 | 3 | 4 | 5 | 6 | 7 | 8 | 9 | 10+

B=BREAKFAST   L=LUNCH   D=DINNER   S=SNACKS   E=EXERCISE

DAY (23)

MO TU WE TH FR SA SU

DATE ....

HOW I FEEL

BREAKFAST	LUNCH	DINNER
....		
....		
....		
....		
....		

SNACKS

....

....

....

TOTAL CALORIES

_____

PROTEIN CONTENT   FIBER CONTENT

_____   _____

OTHER

....

WEIGHT   SLEEP   WATER   PROTEIN

EXERCISE / OTHER ACTIVITIES   SET / REPS / DISTANCE   TIME

....	....	....
....	....	....
....	....	....
....	....	....
....	....	....

NOTES

....

....

 6A 7 8 9 10 11 12P 1 2 3 4 5 6 7 8 9 10+

B=BREAKFAST   L=LUNCH   D=DINNER   S=SNACKS   E=EXERCISE

HOW I FEEL

😃 🙂 😐 ☹️
○ ○ ○ ○

MO TU WE TH FR SA SU

DATE ....

DAY (24)

BREAKFAST	LUNCH	DINNER
....	....	....
....	....	....
....	....	....
....	....	....
....	....	....

SNACKS

....

....

....

TOTAL CALORIES

_____

PROTEIN CONTENT   FIBER CONTENT

WEIGHT   SLEEP   WATER   PROTEIN

OTHER

....

EXERCISE / OTHER ACTIVITIES   SET / REPS / DISTANCE   TIME

....	....	....
....	....	....
....	....	....
....	....	....
....	....	....

NOTES

....

....

6A 7 8 9 10 11 12P 1 2 3 4 5 6 7 8 9 10+

B=BREAKFAST   L=LUNCH   D=DINNER   S=SNACKS   E=EXERCISE

DAY (25)

MO TU WE TH FR SA SU

DATE ....

HOW I FEEL

○ ○ ○ ○

BREAKFAST	LUNCH	DINNER
....	....	....
....	....	....
....	....	....
....	....	....
....	....	....

_____   ____

SNACKS

....

....

....

TOTAL CALORIES

_____

PROTEIN CONTENT   FIBER CONTENT

_____   _____

WEIGHT   SLEEP   WATER   PROTEIN

OTHER

....

♡ EXERCISE / OTHER ACTIVITIES

EXERCISE / OTHER ACTIVITIES	SET / REPS / DISTANCE	TIME
....	....	....
....	....	....
....	....	....
....	....	....
....	....	....

NOTES

....

....

6A 7 8 9 10 11 12P 1 2 3 4 5 6 7 8 9 10+

B=BREAKFAST   L=LUNCH   D=DINNER   S=SNACKS   E=EXERCISE

HOW I FEEL

MO TU WE TH FR SA SU

DATE ....

DAY (26)

BREAKFAST

....
....
....
....
....

SNACKS

....
....
....

TOTAL CALORIES

_____

PROTEIN CONTENT   FIBER CONTENT

_____   _____

OTHER

....

LUNCH

....
....
....
....
....
....
....
....
....
....

DINNER

....
....
....
....
....
....

WEIGHT   SLEEP   WATER   PROTEIN

_____   _____   ....

EXERCISE / OTHER ACTIVITIES   SET / REPS / DISTANCE   TIME

....
....
....
....
....

NOTES

....
....

6A 7 8 9 10 11 12P 1 2 3 4 5 6 7 8 9 10+

B=BREAKFAST   L=LUNCH   D=DINNER   S=SNACKS   E=EXERCISE

DAY (27)

MO TU WE TH FR SA SU

DATE ....

BREAKFAST	LUNCH	DINNER
....	....	....
....	....	....
....	....	....
....	....	....
....	....	....

SNACKS

....

....

....

TOTAL CALORIES

_____

PROTEIN CONTENT   FIBER CONTENT

WEIGHT   SLEEP   WATER   PROTEIN

OTHER

....

♥ **EXERCISE / OTHER ACTIVITIES**   SET / REPS / DISTANCE   TIME

....	....	....
....	....	....
....	....	....
....	....	....
....	....	....

NOTES

....

....

🕐   6A 7 8 9 10 11 12P 1 2 3 4 5 6 7 8 9 10+

B=BREAKFAST   L=LUNCH   D=DINNER   S=SNACKS   E=EXERCISE

HOW I FEEL

😃 🙂 😐 😞
○ ○ ○ ○

MO TU WE TH FR SA SU

DATE ....

DAY (28)

BREAKFAST | LUNCH | DINNER

....
....
....
....
....

SNACKS

....
....
....

TOTAL CALORIES

PROTEIN CONTENT FIBER CONTENT

WEIGHT   SLEEP   WATER   PROTEIN

OTHER

❤ EXERCISE / OTHER ACTIVITIES | SET / REPS / DISTANCE | TIME

....
....
....
....
....

NOTES

....
....

 6A 7 8 9 10 11 12P 1 2 3 4 5 6 7 8 9 10+

B=BREAKFAST L=LUNCH D=DINNER S=SNACKS E=EXERCISE

DAY (29)

MO TU WE TH FR SA SU

DATE ....

HOW I FEEL

○ ○ ○ ○

BREAKFAST	LUNCH	DINNER
....	....	....
....	....	....
....	....	....
....	....	....
....	....	....

SNACKS

....

....

....

TOTAL CALORIES

_____

PROTEIN CONTENT FIBER CONTENT

_____ _____

WEIGHT   **SLEEP**   **WATER**   **PROTEIN**

OTHER

....

❤ **EXERCISE / OTHER ACTIVITIES**   SET / REPS / DISTANCE   TIME

....

....

....

....

....

NOTES

....

....

🕐 6A 7 8 9 10 11 12P 1 2 3 4 5 6 7 8 9 10+

B=BREAKFAST   L=LUNCH   D=DINNER   S=SNACKS   E=EXERCISE

DAY 30

MY MEASUREMENTS

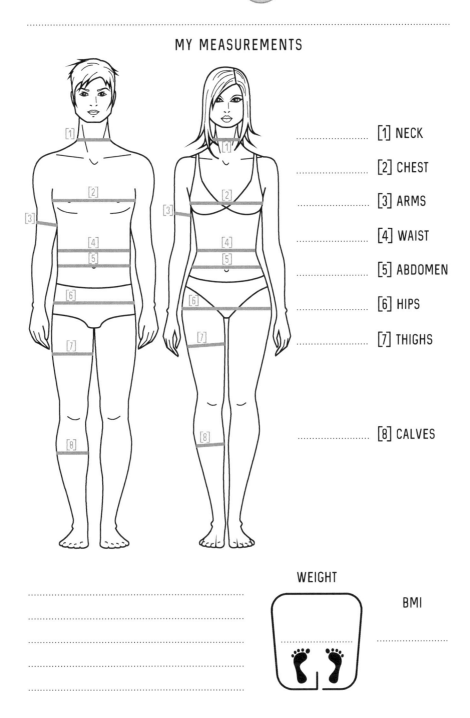

.... [1] NECK

.... [2] CHEST

.... [3] ARMS

.... [4] WAIST

.... [5] ABDOMEN

.... [6] HIPS

.... [7] THIGHS

.... [8] CALVES

WEIGHT

BMI

DAY (30)

MO TU WE TH FR SA SU

DATE ....

HOW I FEEL

○ ○ ○ ○

BREAKFAST

....
....
....
....
....

_____ ___

SNACKS

....
....
....

LUNCH

....
....
....
....
....
....
....
....
....
....

DINNER

....
....
....
....
....
....
....
....

TOTAL CALORIES

_____

PROTEIN CONTENT   FIBER CONTENT

_____ _____

OTHER

....

WEIGHT   SLEEP   WATER   PROTEIN

....

===========

....

♥ EXERCISE / OTHER ACTIVITIES   SET / REPS / DISTANCE   TIME

....
....
....
....
....
....

NOTES

....
....

🕐 6A 7   8   9   10 11 12P 1   2   3   4   5   6   7   8   9   10+

B=BREAKFAST   L=LUNCH   D=DINNER   S=SNACKS   E=EXERCISE

HOW I FEEL

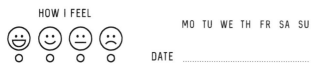

😃 ☺ 😐 ☹
○ ○ ○ ○

MO TU WE TH FR SA SU

DATE ....

DAY (31)

BREAKFAST	LUNCH	DINNER
....	....	....
....	....	....
....	....	....
....	....	....
....	....	....

———————— ——

SNACKS

....
....
....

TOTAL CALORIES

————————————

PROTEIN CONTENT   FIBER CONTENT

———————— ————

OTHER

....

WEIGHT   SLEEP   WATER   PROTEIN

❤ **EXERCISE / OTHER ACTIVITIES**   SET / REPS / DISTANCE   TIME

....	....	....
....	....	....
....	....	....
....	....	....
....	....	....

NOTES

....
....

🕐 6A 7 8 9 10 11 12P 1 2 3 4 5 6 7 8 9 10+

B=BREAKFAST   L=LUNCH   D=DINNER   S=SNACKS   E=EXERCISE

DAY (32)

MO TU WE TH FR SA SU

DATE ....

HOW I FEEL

BREAKFAST	LUNCH	DINNER
....	....	....
....	....	....
....	....	....
....	....	....
....	....	....

SNACKS

....

....

....

TOTAL CALORIES

WEIGHT   SLEEP   WATER   PROTEIN

PROTEIN CONTENT   FIBER CONTENT

OTHER

....

♥ EXERCISE / OTHER ACTIVITIES   SET / REPS / DISTANCE   TIME

....	....	....
....	....	....
....	....	....
....	....	....
....	....	....

NOTES

....

....

🕐   6A   7   8   9   10   11   12P   1   2   3   4   5   6   7   8   9   10+

B=BREAKFAST   L=LUNCH   D=DINNER   S=SNACKS   E=EXERCISE

HOW I FEEL

😃 🙂 😐 ☹️
○ ○ ○ ○

MO TU WE TH FR SA SU

DATE ....

DAY (33)

BREAKFAST	LUNCH	DINNER
....	....	....
....	....	....
....	....	....
....	....	....
....	....	....
	....	....

SNACKS

....
....
....

TOTAL CALORIES

_____

PROTEIN CONTENT FIBER CONTENT

_____ _____

WEIGHT   SLEEP   WATER   PROTEIN

======== ....

OTHER
....

❤️ EXERCISE / OTHER ACTIVITIES   SET / REPS / DISTANCE   TIME

....	....	....
....	....	....
....	....	....
....	....	....
....	....	....

NOTES
....
....

🕐 6A 7 8 9 10 11 12P 1 2 3 4 5 6 7 8 9 10+

B=BREAKFAST   L=LUNCH   D=DINNER   S=SNACKS   E=EXERCISE

DAY (34)

MO TU WE TH FR SA SU

DATE ....

HOW I FEEL

BREAKFAST

....
....
....
....
....

SNACKS

....
....
....

TOTAL CALORIES

_____

PROTEIN CONTENT FIBER CONTENT

_____ _____

OTHER

....

LUNCH

....
....
....
....
....
....
....
....
....
....

DINNER

....
....
....
....
....
....
....
....
....

WEIGHT   SLEEP   WATER   PROTEIN

❤ EXERCISE / OTHER ACTIVITIES   SET / REPS / DISTANCE   TIME

....
....
....
....
....

NOTES

....
....

6A 7 8 9 10 11 12P 1 2 3 4 5 6 7 8 9 10+

B=BREAKFAST   L=LUNCH   D=DINNER   S=SNACKS   E=EXERCISE

HOW I FEEL

😀 😊 😐 😞
○ ○ ○ ○

MO TU WE TH FR SA SU

DATE ....

DAY (35)

BREAKFAST	LUNCH	DINNER
....	....	....
....	....	....
....	....	....
....	....	....
....	....	....

SNACKS

....

....

....

TOTAL CALORIES

_____

PROTEIN CONTENT FIBER CONTENT

_____ _____

OTHER

....

WEIGHT   SLEEP   WATER   PROTEIN

❤ EXERCISE / OTHER ACTIVITIES

	SET / REPS / DISTANCE	TIME
....	....	....
....	....	....
....	....	....
....	....	....
....	....	....

NOTES

....

....

🕐 6A 7 8 9 10 11 12P 1 2 3 4 5 6 7 8 9 10+

B=BREAKFAST   L=LUNCH   D=DINNER   S=SNACKS   E=EXERCISE

DAY (36)

DATE ....

HOW I FEEL

BREAKFAST

....
....
....
....
....

SNACKS

....
....
....

LUNCH

....
....
....
....
....
....
....
....
....
....
....
....

DINNER

....
....
....
....
....
....
....
....
....
....
....
....

TOTAL CALORIES

_____

PROTEIN CONTENT   FIBER CONTENT

_____   _____

WEIGHT   SLEEP   WATER   PROTEIN

_____   ....

OTHER

....

♥ EXERCISE / OTHER ACTIVITIES   SET / REPS / DISTANCE   TIME

....
....
....
....
....

NOTES

....
....

🕐 6A 7 8 9 10 11 12P 1 2 3 4 5 6 7 8 9 10+

B=BREAKFAST   L=LUNCH   D=DINNER   S=SNACKS   E=EXERCISE

HOW I FEEL

😀 ○ 🙂 ○ 😐 ○ ☹ ○

MO TU WE TH FR SA SU

DATE ....

DAY (37)

BREAKFAST	LUNCH	DINNER
....	....	....
....	....	....
....	....	....
....	....	....
....	....	....

_____ ___

SNACKS

....
....
....

TOTAL CALORIES

_____

PROTEIN CONTENT   FIBER CONTENT

_____ _____

WEIGHT   SLEEP   WATER   PROTEIN

OTHER

❤ EXERCISE / OTHER ACTIVITIES

SET / REPS / DISTANCE   TIME

....
....
....
....
....

NOTES

....
....
....

🕐 6A 7 8 9 10 11 12P 1 2 3 4 5 6 7 8 9 10+

B=BREAKFAST   L=LUNCH   D=DINNER   S=SNACKS   E=EXERCISE

DAY (38)

DATE ....

BREAKFAST

....
....
....
....
....

SNACKS

....
....
....
....

TOTAL CALORIES

_____

PROTEIN CONTENT   FIBER CONTENT

_____   _____

OTHER

LUNCH

....
....
....
....
....
....
....
....
....

DINNER

....
....
....
....
....
....
....
....
....

WEIGHT   SLEEP   WATER   PROTEIN

_____   _____   ....

❤ EXERCISE / OTHER ACTIVITIES   SET / REPS / DISTANCE   TIME

....
....
....
....
....

NOTES

....
....

🕐 6A 7 8 9 10 11 12P 1 2 3 4 5 6 7 8 9 10+

B=BREAKFAST   L=LUNCH   D=DINNER   S=SNACKS   E=EXERCISE

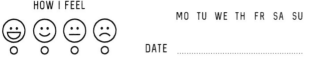

HOW I FEEL

MO TU WE TH FR SA SU

DATE ....

DAY (39)

BREAKFAST

....
....
....
....
....

LUNCH

....
....
....
....
....
....
....
....
....
....
....

DINNER

....
....
....
....
....

SNACKS

....
....
....

TOTAL CALORIES

_____ ____

PROTEIN CONTENT FIBER CONTENT

_____ _____

WEIGHT   **SLEEP**   **WATER**   **PROTEIN**

OTHER

....

❤ EXERCISE / OTHER ACTIVITIES

SET / REPS / DISTANCE   TIME

....
....
....
....
....

NOTES

....
....

🕐 6A 7 8 9 10 11 12P 1 2 3 4 5 6 7 8 9 10+

B=BREAKFAST L=LUNCH D=DINNER S=SNACKS E=EXERCISE

DAY (40)

MO TU WE TH FR SA SU

DATE ....

BREAKFAST

....
....
....
....
....

_____ _____

SNACKS

....
....
....

LUNCH

....
....
....
....
....
....
....
....
....
....
....

DINNER

....
....
....
....
....
....
....
....
....

TOTAL CALORIES

_____

PROTEIN CONTENT   FIBER CONTENT

_____   _____

WEIGHT

SLEEP

WATER

PROTEIN

OTHER

_____ _____ ══════ ══════ ....

....

♥ EXERCISE / OTHER ACTIVITIES

SET / REPS / DISTANCE   TIME

....
....
....
....
....

_____ _____ _____

NOTES

....
....

🕐 6A 7 8 9 10 11 12P 1 2 3 4 5 6 7 8 9 10+

B=BREAKFAST   L=LUNCH   D=DINNER   S=SNACKS   E=EXERCISE

HOW I FEEL

😃 ☺ 😐 ☹

MO TU WE TH FR SA SU

DATE ....

DAY ㊸

BREAKFAST	LUNCH	DINNER
....	....	....
....	....	....
....	....	....
....	....	....
....	....	....

_____ ____

SNACKS

....

....

....

TOTAL CALORIES

_____

PROTEIN CONTENT   FIBER CONTENT

_____ _____

WEIGHT   SLEEP   WATER   PROTEIN

OTHER

....

♥ EXERCISE / OTHER ACTIVITIES   SET / REPS / DISTANCE   TIME

EXERCISE / OTHER ACTIVITIES	SET / REPS / DISTANCE	TIME
....	....	....
....	....	....
....	....	....
....	....	....
....	....	....

NOTES

....

....

🕐 6A 7 8 9 10 11 12P 1 2 3 4 5 6 7 8 9 10+

B=BREAKFAST   L=LUNCH   D=DINNER   S=SNACKS   E=EXERCISE

DAY (42)

MO TU WE TH FR SA SU

DATE ....

HOW I FEEL

BREAKFAST
....
....
....
....
....
_____   _____

LUNCH
....
....
....
....
....
....
....
....
....
....
....
....

DINNER
....
....
....
....
....
....
....
....
....
....
....

SNACKS
....
....
....

TOTAL CALORIES
_____

PROTEIN CONTENT   FIBER CONTENT
_____   _____

OTHER
....

WEIGHT   **SLEEP**   **WATER**   **PROTEIN**

♡ EXERCISE / OTHER ACTIVITIES   SET / REPS / DISTANCE   TIME

....
....
....
....
....

NOTES
....
....

6A 7 8 9 10 11 12P 1 2 3 4 5 6 7 8 9 10+

B=BREAKFAST   L=LUNCH   D=DINNER   S=SNACKS   E=EXERCISE

HOW I FEEL

MO TU WE TH FR SA SU

DATE ....

DAY (43)

BREAKFAST

....
....
....
....
....
_____ _____

SNACKS

....
....
....

TOTAL CALORIES

_____

PROTEIN CONTENT FIBER CONTENT

_____ _____

OTHER

....

LUNCH

....
....
....
....
....
....
....
....
....
....
....

DINNER

....
....
....
....
....
....

WEIGHT	SLEEP	WATER	PROTEIN

EXERCISE / OTHER ACTIVITIES	SET / REPS / DISTANCE	TIME
....	....	....
....	....	....
....	....	....
....	....	....
....	....	....

NOTES

....
....

6A 7 8 9 10 11 12P 1 2 3 4 5 6 7 8 9 10+

B=BREAKFAST   L=LUNCH   D=DINNER   S=SNACKS   E=EXERCISE

DAY (44)

MO TU WE TH FR SA SU

DATE ....

HOW I FEEL

BREAKFAST	LUNCH	DINNER
....	....	....
....	....	....
....	....	....
....	....	....
....	....	....

SNACKS

....

....

....

TOTAL CALORIES

_____ ____

PROTEIN CONTENT   FIBER CONTENT

_____ _____

WEIGHT   SLEEP   WATER   PROTEIN

OTHER

....

♥ EXERCISE / OTHER ACTIVITIES   SET / REPS / DISTANCE   TIME

....	....	....
....	....	....
....	....	....
....	....	....
....	....	....

NOTES

....

....

🕐 6A 7 8 9 10 11 12P 1 2 3 4 5 6 7 8 9 10+

B=BREAKFAST   L=LUNCH   D=DINNER   S=SNACKS   E=EXERCISE

HOW I FEEL

😄 😊 😐 😞
○ ○ ○ ○

MO TU WE TH FR SA SU

DATE ....

DAY 45

BREAKFAST

LUNCH

DINNER

SNACKS

TOTAL CALORIES

WEIGHT   SLEEP   WATER   PROTEIN

PROTEIN CONTENT FIBER CONTENT

OTHER

EXERCISE / OTHER ACTIVITIES   SET / REPS / DISTANCE   TIME

NOTES

6A 7 8 9 10 11 12P 1 2 3 4 5 6 7 8 9 10+

B=BREAKFAST   L=LUNCH   D=DINNER   S=SNACKS   E=EXERCISE

DAY (46)

MO TU WE TH FR SA SU

DATE ....

HOW I FEEL

BREAKFAST
....
....
....
....
....
_____ _____

SNACKS
....
....
....
....

TOTAL CALORIES
_____

PROTEIN CONTENT FIBER CONTENT
_____ _____

OTHER
....

LUNCH
....
....
....
....
....
....
....
....
....
....
_____ _____

DINNER
....
....
....
....
....
....
....
....
....
....
....
_____ _____

WEIGHT   SLEEP   WATER   PROTEIN
_____   _____   ....

EXERCISE / OTHER ACTIVITIES	SET / REPS / DISTANCE	TIME
....	....	....
....	....	....
....	....	....
....	....	....
....	....	....

NOTES
....
....

6A 7 8 9 10 11 12P 1 2 3 4 5 6 7 8 9 10+

B=BREAKFAST   L=LUNCH   D=DINNER   S=SNACKS   E=EXERCISE

HOW I FEEL

😄 🙂 😐 🙁
○ ○ ○ ○

MO TU WE TH FR SA SU

DATE ....

DAY (47)

BREAKFAST	LUNCH	DINNER
....	....	....
....	....	....
....	....	....
....	....	....
....	....	....
....	....	....

SNACKS

....

....

....

TOTAL CALORIES

_____

PROTEIN CONTENT   FIBER CONTENT

_____   _____

OTHER

WEIGHT   SLEEP   WATER   PROTEIN

_____   _____   ....

....

♡ EXERCISE / OTHER ACTIVITIES   SET / REPS / DISTANCE   TIME

....	....	....
....	....	....
....	....	....
....	....	....
....	....	....

NOTES

....

....

🕐 6A 7 8 9 10 11 12P 1 2 3 4 5 6 7 8 9 10+

B=BREAKFAST   L=LUNCH   D=DINNER   S=SNACKS   E=EXERCISE

DAY (48)

MO TU WE TH FR SA SU

DATE ....

HOW I FEEL

BREAKFAST

....
....
....
....
....

SNACKS

....
....
....

TOTAL CALORIES

_____

PROTEIN CONTENT   FIBER CONTENT

_____   _____

OTHER

....

LUNCH

....
....
....
....
....
....
....
....
....

DINNER

....
....
....
....
....
....
....
....
....

WEIGHT   **SLEEP**   **WATER**   **PROTEIN**

EXERCISE / OTHER ACTIVITIES   SET / REPS / DISTANCE   TIME

....
....
....
....
....

NOTES

....
....
....

6A 7 8 9 10 11 12P 1 2 3 4 5 6 7 8 9 10+

B=BREAKFAST   L=LUNCH   D=DINNER   S=SNACKS   E=EXERCISE

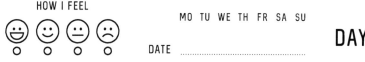

HOW I FEEL

MO TU WE TH FR SA SU

DATE ....

DAY 49

BREAKFAST

LUNCH

DINNER

SNACKS

TOTAL CALORIES

PROTEIN CONTENT   FIBER CONTENT

WEIGHT

SLEEP

WATER

PROTEIN

OTHER

EXERCISE / OTHER ACTIVITIES   SET / REPS / DISTANCE   TIME

NOTES

6A 7   8   9   10 11 12P 1   2   3   4   5   6   7   8   9   10+

B=BREAKFAST   L=LUNCH   D=DINNER   S=SNACKS   E=EXERCISE

DAY

MO TU WE TH FR SA SU

DATE ....

HOW I FEEL

BREAKFAST   LUNCH   DINNER

....
....
....
....
....

SNACKS

....
....
....

TOTAL CALORIES

_____

PROTEIN CONTENT FIBER CONTENT

WEIGHT   SLEEP   WATER   PROTEIN

_____ _____   ========   ....

OTHER

....

♡ EXERCISE / OTHER ACTIVITIES   SET / REPS / DISTANCE   TIME

....
....
....
....
....

NOTES

....
....

6A 7 8 9 10 11 12P 1 2 3 4 5 6 7 8 9 10+

B=BREAKFAST   L=LUNCH   D=DINNER   S=SNACKS   E=EXERCISE

HOW I FEEL

😃 ○ 🙂 ○ 😐 ○ 🙁 ○

MO TU WE TH FR SA SU

DATE ....

DAY (51)

BREAKFAST	LUNCH	DINNER
....	....	....
....	....	....
....	....	....
....	....	....
....	....	....

SNACKS

....
....
....

TOTAL CALORIES

_____

PROTEIN CONTENT FIBER CONTENT

_____ _____

WEIGHT SLEEP WATER PROTEIN

OTHER ....

❤ EXERCISE / OTHER ACTIVITIES   SET / REPS / DISTANCE   TIME

....	....	....
....	....	....
....	....	....
....	....	....
....	....	....

NOTES

....
....

🕐 6A 7 8 9 10 11 12P 1 2 3 4 5 6 7 8 9 10+

B=BREAKFAST L=LUNCH D=DINNER S=SNACKS E=EXERCISE

DAY (52)

DATE ....

HOW I FEEL

BREAKFAST   LUNCH   DINNER

....
....
....
....
....
_____

SNACKS

....
....
....

TOTAL CALORIES

_____

PROTEIN CONTENT   FIBER CONTENT

WEIGHT   SLEEP   WATER   PROTEIN

_____   _____   ========   ....

OTHER

....

EXERCISE / OTHER ACTIVITIES   SET / REPS / DISTANCE   TIME

....
....
....
....
....

NOTES

....
....

6A 7 8 9 10 11 12P 1 2 3 4 5 6 7 8 9 10+

B=BREAKFAST   L=LUNCH   D=DINNER   S=SNACKS   E=EXERCISE

HOW I FEEL

MO TU WE TH FR SA SU

DATE ....

DAY (53)

BREAKFAST

....
....
....
....
....

SNACKS

....
....
....

TOTAL CALORIES

_____

PROTEIN CONTENT FIBER CONTENT

_____   _____

OTHER

LUNCH

....
....
....
....
....
....
....
....
....
....
....

DINNER

....
....
....
....
....
....
....
....

WEIGHT   SLEEP   WATER   PROTEIN

_____   _____   ....

....

♥ EXERCISE / OTHER ACTIVITIES   SET / REPS / DISTANCE   TIME

.... | .... | ....
.... | .... | ....
.... | .... | ....
.... | .... | ....
.... | .... | ....

NOTES

....
....

🕐 6A 7 8 9 10 11 12P 1 2 3 4 5 6 7 8 9 10+

B=BREAKFAST L=LUNCH D=DINNER S=SNACKS E=EXERCISE

DAY 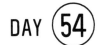 54

MO TU WE TH FR SA SU

DATE ....

HOW I FEEL

BREAKFAST	LUNCH	DINNER

SNACKS

TOTAL CALORIES

PROTEIN CONTENT   FIBER CONTENT

WEIGHT   SLEEP   WATER   PROTEIN

OTHER
....

♥ EXERCISE / OTHER ACTIVITIES	SET / REPS / DISTANCE	TIME

NOTES
....
....
....

6A 7 8 9 10 11 12P 1 2 3 4 5 6 7 8 9 10+

B=BREAKFAST   L=LUNCH   D=DINNER   S=SNACKS   E=EXERCISE

HOW I FEEL

😃 🙂 😐 🙁
○ ○ ○ ○

MO TU WE TH FR SA SU

DATE ....

DAY (55)

BREAKFAST	LUNCH	DINNER
....	....	....
....	....	....
....	....	....
....	....	....
....	....	....

SNACKS

....

....

....

TOTAL CALORIES

_____

PROTEIN CONTENT   FIBER CONTENT

_____ _____

OTHER

WEIGHT   SLEEP   WATER   PROTEIN

....

❤ EXERCISE / OTHER ACTIVITIES

SET / REPS / DISTANCE   TIME

NOTES

....

....

🕐 6A 7 8 9 10 11 12P 1 2 3 4 5 6 7 8 9 10+

B=BREAKFAST   L=LUNCH   D=DINNER   S=SNACKS   E=EXERCISE

DAY (56)

MO TU WE TH FR SA SU

DATE ....

HOW I FEEL

○ ○ ○ ○

BREAKFAST	LUNCH	DINNER
....	....	....
....	....	....
....	....	....
....	....	....
....	....	....

SNACKS

....

....

....

....

TOTAL CALORIES

_____

PROTEIN CONTENT FIBER CONTENT

_____ _____

OTHER

....

WEIGHT   SLEEP   WATER   PROTEIN

❤ EXERCISE / OTHER ACTIVITIES	SET / REPS / DISTANCE	TIME
....	
....	
....	
....	
....	

NOTES

....

....

6A 7 8 9 10 11 12P 1 2 3 4 5 6 7 8 9 10+

B=BREAKFAST   L=LUNCH   D=DINNER   S=SNACKS   E=EXERCISE

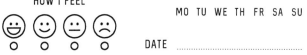

BREAKFAST

....
....
....
....
....
_____ ___

SNACKS

....
....
....
_____ ___

TOTAL CALORIES

_____

PROTEIN CONTENT FIBER CONTENT

_____ _____

OTHER

LUNCH

....
....
....
....
....
....
....
....
....
....
....

DINNER

....
....
....
....
....
....
....
....

WEIGHT   SLEEP   WATER   PROTEIN

EXERCISE / OTHER ACTIVITIES   SET / REPS / DISTANCE   TIME

....
....
....
....
....

NOTES

....
....
....

6A 7 8 9 10 11 12P 1 2 3 4 5 6 7 8 9 10+

B=BREAKFAST L=LUNCH D=DINNER S=SNACKS E=EXERCISE

DAY (58)

DATE ....

HOW I FEEL

 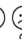

BREAKFAST	LUNCH	DINNER
....	....	....
....	....	....
....	....	....
....	....	....
....	....	....

SNACKS

....

....

....

TOTAL CALORIES

_____

PROTEIN CONTENT   FIBER CONTENT

_____ _____

OTHER

WEIGHT   SLEEP   WATER   PROTEIN

♡ EXERCISE / OTHER ACTIVITIES   SET / REPS / DISTANCE   TIME

....

....

....

....

NOTES

....

....

6A 7 8 9 10 11 12P 1 2 3 4 5 6 7 8 9 10+

B=BREAKFAST   L=LUNCH   D=DINNER   S=SNACKS   E=EXERCISE

HOW I FEEL

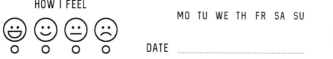

MO TU WE TH FR SA SU

DATE ....

DAY 59

BREAKFAST

....
....
....
....
....
_____ ____

SNACKS

....
....
....
_____ ____

TOTAL CALORIES

_____

PROTEIN CONTENT FIBER CONTENT

_____ _____

OTHER

....

LUNCH

....
....
....
....
....
....
....
....
....
....
....
....

WEIGHT   **SLEEP**   **WATER**   **PROTEIN**

==========   ==========   ....

DINNER

....
....
....
....
....
....
....
....

EXERCISE / OTHER ACTIVITIES	SET / REPS / DISTANCE	TIME
....	....	....
....	....	....
....	....	....
....	....	....
....	....	....

NOTES

....
....

6A 7 8 9 10 11 12P 1 2 3 4 5 6 7 8 9 10+

B=BREAKFAST L=LUNCH D=DINNER S=SNACKS E=EXERCISE

DAY 60

MY MEASUREMENTS

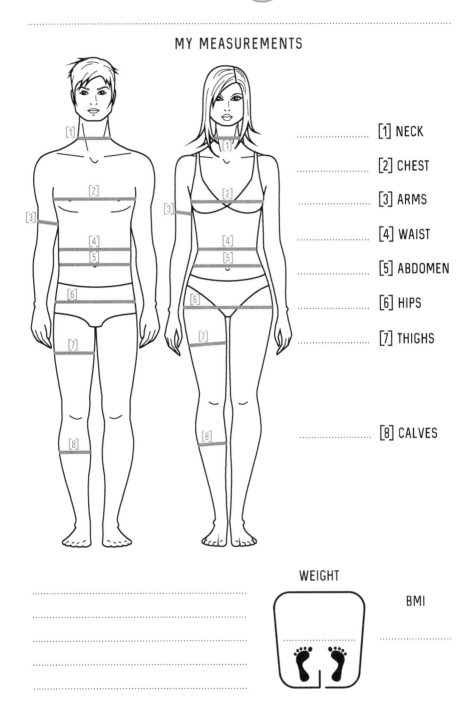

.... [1] NECK

.... [2] CHEST

.... [3] ARMS

.... [4] WAIST

.... [5] ABDOMEN

.... [6] HIPS

.... [7] THIGHS

.... [8] CALVES

WEIGHT

BMI

HOW I FEEL

☺ ☺ ☺ ☹
○ ○ ○ ○

MO TU WE TH FR SA SU

DATE ....

DAY 60

BREAKFAST

....
....
....
....
....

SNACKS

....
....
....

TOTAL CALORIES

_____

PROTEIN CONTENT   FIBER CONTENT

_____ _____

LUNCH

....
....
....
....
....
....
....
....
....
....
....
....

DINNER

....
....
....
....
....
....
....
....
....
....
....

WEIGHT   SLEEP   WATER   PROTEIN

OTHER

❤ EXERCISE / OTHER ACTIVITIES   SET / REPS / DISTANCE   TIME

....
....
....
....
....

NOTES

....
....
....

🕐 6A 7 8 9 10 11 12P 1 2 3 4 5 6 7 8 9 10+

B=BREAKFAST   L=LUNCH   D=DINNER   S=SNACKS   E=EXERCISE

DAY

MO TU WE TH FR SA SU

DATE ....

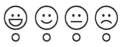

HOW I FEEL

BREAKFAST	LUNCH	DINNER

....

SNACKS

....

TOTAL CALORIES

....

PROTEIN CONTENT FIBER CONTENT

OTHER

....

WEIGHT   SLEEP   WATER   PROTEIN

♡ EXERCISE / OTHER ACTIVITIES   SET / REPS / DISTANCE   TIME

....

NOTES

....

6A 7 8 9 10 11 12P 1 2 3 4 5 6 7 8 9 10+

B=BREAKFAST   L=LUNCH   D=DINNER   S=SNACKS   E=EXERCISE

HOW I FEEL

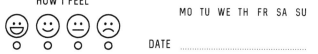

MO TU WE TH FR SA SU

DATE ....

DAY 62

BREAKFAST

....
....
....
....
....

SNACKS

....
....
....

TOTAL CALORIES

_____

PROTEIN CONTENT   FIBER CONTENT

_____   _____

OTHER

LUNCH

....
....
....
....
....
....
....
....
....
....
....

DINNER

....
....
....
....
....
....
....
....
....

WEIGHT   SLEEP   WATER   PROTEIN

_____   _____   ....

EXERCISE / OTHER ACTIVITIES

SET / REPS / DISTANCE   TIME

....
....
....
....
....

NOTES

....
....
....

6A 7 8 9 10 11 12P 1 2 3 4 5 6 7 8 9 10+

B=BREAKFAST   L=LUNCH   D=DINNER   S=SNACKS   E=EXERCISE

DAY

HOW I FEEL

BREAKFAST | LUNCH | DINNER

....

....

....

....

....

SNACKS

....

....

....

TOTAL CALORIES

WEIGHT   SLEEP   WATER   PROTEIN

PROTEIN CONTENT   FIBER CONTENT

OTHER

....

♥ EXERCISE / OTHER ACTIVITIES   SET / REPS / DISTANCE   TIME

....

....

....

....

....

NOTES

....

....

🕐 6A 7 8 9 10 11 12P 1 2 3 4 5 6 7 8 9 10+

B=BREAKFAST   L=LUNCH   D=DINNER   S=SNACKS   E=EXERCISE

HOW I FEEL

MO TU WE TH FR SA SU

DATE ....

DAY (64)

BREAKFAST

LUNCH

DINNER

SNACKS

TOTAL CALORIES

PROTEIN CONTENT   FIBER CONTENT

WEIGHT   SLEEP   WATER   PROTEIN

OTHER

♥ EXERCISE / OTHER ACTIVITIES   SET / REPS / DISTANCE   TIME

NOTES

6A 7 8 9 10 11 12P 1 2 3 4 5 6 7 8 9 10+

B=BREAKFAST   L=LUNCH   D=DINNER   S=SNACKS   E=EXERCISE

DAY 65

MO TU WE TH FR SA SU

DATE ....

BREAKFAST	LUNCH	DINNER
....	....	....
....	....	....
....	....	....
....	....	....
....	....	....
_____	....	....

SNACKS

....
....
....

TOTAL CALORIES

_____

PROTEIN CONTENT   FIBER CONTENT

_____ _____

WEIGHT   SLEEP   WATER   PROTEIN

==================== ....

OTHER

....

♥ EXERCISE / OTHER ACTIVITIES

EXERCISE / OTHER ACTIVITIES	SET / REPS / DISTANCE	TIME
....	....	....
....	....	....
....	....	....
....	....	....
....	....	....

NOTES

....
....

🕐   6A 7 8 9 10 11 12P 1 2 3 4 5 6 7 8 9 10+

B=BREAKFAST   L=LUNCH   D=DINNER   S=SNACKS   E=EXERCISE

HOW I FEEL

☺ ☺ ☺ ☹
○ ○ ○ ○

MO TU WE TH FR SA SU

DATE ....

DAY 66

BREAKFAST	LUNCH	DINNER
....	....	....
....	....	....
....	....	....
....	....	....
....	....	....

SNACKS

....
....
....

TOTAL CALORIES

_____

PROTEIN CONTENT   FIBER CONTENT

WEIGHT   SLEEP   WATER   PROTEIN

OTHER ....

♥ EXERCISE / OTHER ACTIVITIES   SET / REPS / DISTANCE   TIME

....	....	....
....	....	....
....	....	....
....	....	....
....	....	....

NOTES

....
....
....

🕐 6A 7 8 9 10 11 12P 1 2 3 4 5 6 7 8 9 10+

B=BREAKFAST   L=LUNCH   D=DINNER   S=SNACKS   E=EXERCISE

DAY (67)

MO TU WE TH FR SA SU

DATE ....

HOW I FEEL

😀 ○   🙂 ○   😐 ○   🙁 ○

BREAKFAST

LUNCH

DINNER

SNACKS

TOTAL CALORIES

WEIGHT   SLEEP   WATER   PROTEIN

PROTEIN CONTENT   FIBER CONTENT

OTHER

EXERCISE / OTHER ACTIVITIES

SET / REPS / DISTANCE   TIME

NOTES

6A   7   8   9   10   11   12P   1   2   3   4   5   6   7   8   9   10+

B=BREAKFAST   L=LUNCH   D=DINNER   S=SNACKS   E=EXERCISE

HOW I FEEL

:smiley: :smile: :neutral: :frowning:
○   ○   ○   ○

MO TU WE TH FR SA SU

DATE ....

DAY (68)

BREAKFAST

....
....
....
....
....

SNACKS

....
....
....

TOTAL CALORIES

_____

PROTEIN CONTENT   FIBER CONTENT

_____   _____

LUNCH

....
....
....
....
....
....
....
....
....
....
....

DINNER

....
....
....
....
....
....
....
....
....
....
....

WEIGHT   SLEEP   WATER   PROTEIN

OTHER

....

♡ EXERCISE / OTHER ACTIVITIES

SET / REPS / DISTANCE   TIME

....
....
....
....
....

NOTES

....
....
....

🕒 6A 7 8 9 10 11 12P 1 2 3 4 5 6 7 8 9 10+

B=BREAKFAST   L=LUNCH   D=DINNER   S=SNACKS   E=EXERCISE

DAY 69

MO TU WE TH FR SA SU

DATE ....

HOW I FEEL

BREAKFAST

....
....
....
....
....
_____   _____

SNACKS

....
....
....

TOTAL CALORIES
_____

PROTEIN CONTENT   FIBER CONTENT
_____   _____

OTHER
....

LUNCH

....
....
....
....
....
....
....
....
....
....
....

WEIGHT   **SLEEP**   **WATER**   **PROTEIN**

=====================   ....

DINNER

....
....
....
....
....
....
....
....
....
....
....

♥ EXERCISE / OTHER ACTIVITIES

	SET / REPS / DISTANCE	TIME
....	....	....
....	....	....
....	....	....
....	....	....
....	....	....

NOTES
....
....
....

6A 7 8 9 10 11 12P 1 2 3 4 5 6 7 8 9 10+

B=BREAKFAST   L=LUNCH   D=DINNER   S=SNACKS   E=EXERCISE

HOW I FEEL

☺ ☺ ☺ ☹

MO TU WE TH FR SA SU

DATE ....

DAY (70)

BREAKFAST

....
....
....
....
....
_____ ____

SNACKS

....
....
....
_____ ____

LUNCH

....
....
....
....
....
....
....
....
....
....
....
....

DINNER

....
....
....
....
....
....
....
....
....
_____

TOTAL CALORIES

_____

PROTEIN CONTENT   FIBER CONTENT

_____ _____

WEIGHT   SLEEP   WATER   PROTEIN

OTHER ....

♥ EXERCISE / OTHER ACTIVITIES

EXERCISE / OTHER ACTIVITIES	SET / REPS / DISTANCE	TIME
....	....	....
....	....	....
....	....	....
....	....	....
....	....	....

NOTES

....
....

🕐 6A 7 8 9 10 11 12P 1 2 3 4 5 6 7 8 9 10+

B=BREAKFAST   L=LUNCH   D=DINNER   S=SNACKS   E=EXERCISE

DAY

MO TU WE TH FR SA SU

DATE ....

HOW I FEEL

BREAKFAST	LUNCH	DINNER
....	....	....
....	....	....
....	....	....
....	....	....
....	....	....
	....	....

SNACKS

....

....

....

TOTAL CALORIES

_____

PROTEIN CONTENT   FIBER CONTENT

_____   _____

OTHER

....

WEIGHT   SLEEP   WATER   PROTEIN

EXERCISE / OTHER ACTIVITIES   SET / REPS / DISTANCE   TIME

....	....	....
....	....	....
....	....	....
....	....	....
....	....	....

NOTES

....

....

6A   7   8   9   10   11   12P   1   2   3   4   5   6   7   8   9   10+

B=BREAKFAST   L=LUNCH   D=DINNER   S=SNACKS   E=EXERCISE

HOW I FEEL

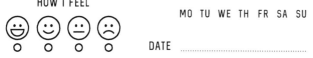

MO TU WE TH FR SA SU

DATE ....

DAY (72)

BREAKFAST	LUNCH	DINNER
....	....	....
....	....	....
....	....	....
....	....	....
....	....	....

SNACKS

....

....

....

TOTAL CALORIES

WEIGHT   SLEEP   WATER   PROTEIN

PROTEIN CONTENT   FIBER CONTENT

OTHER ....

❤ EXERCISE / OTHER ACTIVITIES

	SET / REPS / DISTANCE	TIME
....	....	....
....	....	....
....	....	....
....	....	....
....	....	....

NOTES

....

....

🕐 6A 7 8 9 10 11 12P 1 2 3 4 5 6 7 8 9 10+

B=BREAKFAST   L=LUNCH   D=DINNER   S=SNACKS   E=EXERCISE

DAY (73)

DATE MO TU WE TH FR SA SU

....

BREAKFAST

....
....
....
....
....
_____ ___

LUNCH

....
....
....
....
....
....
....
....
....

DINNER

....
....
....
....
....

SNACKS

....
....
....

TOTAL CALORIES

_____ ___

PROTEIN CONTENT FIBER CONTENT

_____ _____ ____

WEIGHT   SLEEP   WATER   PROTEIN

_____ _____ ....

OTHER
....

❤ EXERCISE / OTHER ACTIVITIES   SET / REPS / DISTANCE   TIME

....
....
....
....
....

NOTES

....
....

6A 7 8 9 10 11 12P 1 2 3 4 5 6 7 8 9 10+

B=BREAKFAST   L=LUNCH   D=DINNER   S=SNACKS   E=EXERCISE

HOW I FEEL

😃 😊 😐 ☹️
○   ○   ○   ○

MO TU WE TH FR SA SU

DATE ....

DAY 74

BREAKFAST	LUNCH	DINNER

SNACKS

TOTAL CALORIES

PROTEIN CONTENT FIBER CONTENT

WEIGHT   SLEEP   WATER   PROTEIN

OTHER

....

♥ EXERCISE / OTHER ACTIVITIES   SET / REPS / DISTANCE   TIME

NOTES

....

....

🕐 6A 7 8 9 10 11 12P 1 2 3 4 5 6 7 8 9 10+

B=BREAKFAST   L=LUNCH   D=DINNER   S=SNACKS   E=EXERCISE

DAY (75)

DATE ....

HOW I FEEL

BREAKFAST

LUNCH

DINNER

....
....
....
....
....

SNACKS

....
....
....

TOTAL CALORIES

_____

PROTEIN CONTENT FIBER CONTENT

_____ _____

OTHER

WEIGHT

SLEEP

WATER

PROTEIN

EXERCISE / OTHER ACTIVITIES

SET / REPS / DISTANCE

TIME

NOTES

6A 7 8 9 10 11 12P 1 2 3 4 5 6 7 8 9 10+

B=BREAKFAST   L=LUNCH   D=DINNER   S=SNACKS   E=EXERCISE

HOW I FEEL

😃 ☺ 😐 ☹
○   ○   ○   ○

MO TU WE TH FR SA SU

DATE ....

DAY (76)

BREAKFAST

....
....
....
....
....
_____ ___

SNACKS

....
....
....
_____ ___

LUNCH

....
....
....
....
....
....
....
....
....
....
....
....

DINNER

....
....
....
....
....
....
....
....
....
_____ ___

TOTAL CALORIES

_____

PROTEIN CONTENT   FIBER CONTENT

_____ _____

OTHER

....

WEIGHT   SLEEP   WATER   PROTEIN

.... ===== ....

❤ EXERCISE / OTHER ACTIVITIES

EXERCISE / OTHER ACTIVITIES	SET / REPS / DISTANCE	TIME
....	....	....
....	....	....
....	....	....
....	....	....
....	....	....

NOTES

....
....
....

🕐 6A 7 8 9 10 11 12P 1 2 3 4 5 6 7 8 9 10+

B=BREAKFAST L=LUNCH D=DINNER S=SNACKS E=EXERCISE

DAY

MO TU WE TH FR SA SU

DATE ....

BREAKFAST

....
....
....
....
....
_____ _____

SNACKS

....
....
....
_____ _____

LUNCH

....
....
....
....
....
....
....
....
....
....
....

DINNER

....
....
....
....
....
....
....
....
....
....
....

TOTAL CALORIES

_____

PROTEIN CONTENT FIBER CONTENT

_____ _____ _____

OTHER

....

WEIGHT   SLEEP   WATER   PROTEIN

====================== ....

♥ EXERCISE / OTHER ACTIVITIES

	SET / REPS / DISTANCE	TIME
....	....	....
....	....	....
....	....	....
....	....	....
....	....	....

NOTES

....
....

6A 7 8 9 10 11 12P 1 2 3 4 5 6 7 8 9 10+

B=BREAKFAST   L=LUNCH   D=DINNER   S=SNACKS   E=EXERCISE

HOW I FEEL

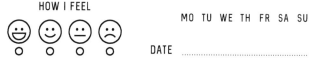

MO TU WE TH FR SA SU

DATE ....

DAY (78)

BREAKFAST

....
....
....
....
....

_____ ____

SNACKS

....
....
....

_____ ____

TOTAL CALORIES

_____

PROTEIN CONTENT FIBER CONTENT

_____ ____

OTHER

....

LUNCH

....
....
....
....
....
....
....
....
....
....
....

DINNER

....
....
....
....
....

_____ ____

WEIGHT SLEEP WATER PROTEIN

_____ _____ ....

♥ EXERCISE / OTHER ACTIVITIES   SET / REPS / DISTANCE   TIME

....
....
....
....
....

NOTES

....
....

🕒 6A 7 8 9 10 11 12P 1 2 3 4 5 6 7 8 9 10+

B=BREAKFAST L=LUNCH D=DINNER S=SNACKS E=EXERCISE

DAY (79)

MO TU WE TH FR SA SU

DATE ....

HOW I FEEL

BREAKFAST	LUNCH	DINNER

SNACKS

TOTAL CALORIES

WEIGHT   SLEEP   WATER   PROTEIN

PROTEIN CONTENT   FIBER CONTENT

OTHER

 EXERCISE / OTHER ACTIVITIES   SET / REPS / DISTANCE   TIME

NOTES

6A 7 8 9 10 11 12P 1 2 3 4 5 6 7 8 9 10+

B=BREAKFAST   L=LUNCH   D=DINNER   S=SNACKS   E=EXERCISE

HOW I FEEL

MO TU WE TH FR SA SU

DATE ....

DAY (80)

BREAKFAST   LUNCH   DINNER

....
....
....
....
....
                   ....
SNACKS   ....
....
....
....
                   ....

TOTAL CALORIES

WEIGHT   SLEEP   WATER   PROTEIN

PROTEIN CONTENT FIBER CONTENT

OTHER
....

♡ EXERCISE / OTHER ACTIVITIES   SET / REPS / DISTANCE   TIME

....
....
....
....
....

NOTES
....
....

 6A 7 8 9 10 11 12P 1 2 3 4 5 6 7 8 9 10+

B=BREAKFAST   L=LUNCH   D=DINNER   S=SNACKS   E=EXERCISE

DAY (81)

MO TU WE TH FR SA SU

DATE ....

HOW I FEEL

BREAKFAST   LUNCH   DINNER

....
....
....
....
....
_____ __   ....

SNACKS

....
....
....

TOTAL CALORIES

_____ __

PROTEIN CONTENT FIBER CONTENT

_____ _____ _____

OTHER

....

WEIGHT   SLEEP   WATER   PROTEIN

❤ EXERCISE / OTHER ACTIVITIES   SET / REPS / DISTANCE   TIME

....
....
....
....
....

NOTES

....
....
....

6A   7   8   9   10   11   12P   1   2   3   4   5   6   7   8   9   10+

B=BREAKFAST   L=LUNCH   D=DINNER   S=SNACKS   E=EXERCISE

HOW I FEEL

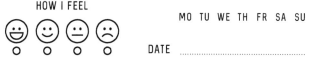

MO TU WE TH FR SA SU

DATE ....

DAY (82)

BREAKFAST	LUNCH	DINNER
....	....	....
....	....	....
....	....	....
....	....	....
....	....	....

SNACKS

....

....

....

TOTAL CALORIES

_____

PROTEIN CONTENT   FIBER CONTENT

_____   _____

OTHER

WEIGHT   SLEEP   WATER   PROTEIN

....

♥ **EXERCISE / OTHER ACTIVITIES**   SET / REPS / DISTANCE   TIME

....	....	....
....	....	....
....	....	....
....	....	....
....	....	....

NOTES

....

....

🕐 6A 7 8 9 10 11 12P 1 2 3 4 5 6 7 8 9 10+

B=BREAKFAST   L=LUNCH   D=DINNER   S=SNACKS   E=EXERCISE

DAY (83)

DATE MO TU WE TH FR SA SU
....

HOW I FEEL

BREAKFAST	LUNCH	DINNER
....	....	....
....	....	....
....	....	....
....	....	....
....	....	....

SNACKS

....

....

....

TOTAL CALORIES

PROTEIN CONTENT   FIBER CONTENT

WEIGHT   SLEEP   WATER   PROTEIN

OTHER
....

❤ EXERCISE / OTHER ACTIVITIES   SET / REPS / DISTANCE   TIME

.... | .... | ....
.... | .... | ....
.... | .... | ....
.... | .... | ....
.... | .... | ....

NOTES
....

....

🕐 6A 7 8 9 10 11 12P 1 2 3 4 5 6 7 8 9 10+

B=BREAKFAST   L=LUNCH   D=DINNER   S=SNACKS   E=EXERCISE

HOW I FEEL

☺ ☺ 😐 ☹

MO TU WE TH FR SA SU

DATE ....

DAY (84)

BREAKFAST

....
....
....
....
....

_____ ____

SNACKS

....
....
....

_____ ____

TOTAL CALORIES

_____

PROTEIN CONTENT FIBER CONTENT

_____ _____

OTHER

....

LUNCH

....
....
....
....
....
....
....
....
....
....
....

DINNER

....
....
....
....
....
....
....
....
....

_____ ____

WEIGHT   SLEEP   WATER   PROTEIN

_____ _____ ....

♡ EXERCISE / OTHER ACTIVITIES

EXERCISE / OTHER ACTIVITIES	SET / REPS / DISTANCE	TIME
....	....	....
....	....	....
....	....	....
....	....	....
....	....	....

NOTES

....
....

🕐 6A 7 8 9 10 11 12P 1 2 3 4 5 6 7 8 9 10+

B=BREAKFAST   L=LUNCH   D=DINNER   S=SNACKS   E=EXERCISE

DAY

MO TU WE TH FR SA SU

DATE ....

BREAKFAST	LUNCH	DINNER
....	....	....
....	....	....
....	....	....
....	....	....
....	....	....

SNACKS

....

....

....

TOTAL CALORIES

WEIGHT   SLEEP   WATER   PROTEIN

PROTEIN CONTENT   FIBER CONTENT

OTHER

....

♥ EXERCISE / OTHER ACTIVITIES

	SET / REPS / DISTANCE	TIME
....		
....		
....		
....		
....		

NOTES

....

....

6A 7 8 9 10 11 12P 1 2 3 4 5 6 7 8 9 10+

B=BREAKFAST   L=LUNCH   D=DINNER   S=SNACKS   E=EXERCISE

HOW I FEEL

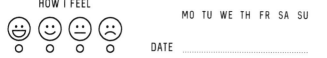

MO TU WE TH FR SA SU

DATE ....

DAY (86)

BREAKFAST	LUNCH	DINNER
....	....	....
....	....	....
....	....	....
....	....	....
....	....	....

SNACKS

....

....

....

TOTAL CALORIES

_____

PROTEIN CONTENT   FIBER CONTENT

_____   _____

WEIGHT   SLEEP   WATER   PROTEIN

_____   _____   =========   ....

OTHER

....

♥ EXERCISE / OTHER ACTIVITIES   SET / REPS / DISTANCE   TIME

....	....	....
....	....	....
....	....	....
....	....	....
....	....	....

NOTES

....

....

🕐 6A 7 8 9 10 11 12P 1 2 3 4 5 6 7 8 9 10+

B=BREAKFAST   L=LUNCH   D=DINNER   S=SNACKS   E=EXERCISE

DAY (87)

MO TU WE TH FR SA SU

DATE ....

BREAKFAST

....
....
....
....
....

SNACKS

....
....
....

LUNCH

....
....
....
....
....
....
....
....
....
....
....

DINNER

....
....
....
....
....
....
....
....
....

TOTAL CALORIES

_____

PROTEIN CONTENT   FIBER CONTENT

_____   _____

OTHER

....

WEIGHT   SLEEP   WATER   PROTEIN

....

♡ EXERCISE / OTHER ACTIVITIES   SET / REPS / DISTANCE   TIME

....
....
....
....
....

NOTES

....
....
....

6A 7 8 9 10 11 12P 1 2 3 4 5 6 7 8 9 10+

B=BREAKFAST   L=LUNCH   D=DINNER   S=SNACKS   E=EXERCISE

HOW I FEEL

😀 ○ 🙂 ○ 😐 ○ ☹ ○

MO TU WE TH FR SA SU

DATE ....

DAY (88)

BREAKFAST

LUNCH

DINNER

....
....
....
....
....

SNACKS

....
....
....

TOTAL CALORIES

_____

PROTEIN CONTENT   FIBER CONTENT

WEIGHT   SLEEP   WATER   PROTEIN

OTHER

....

❤ **EXERCISE / OTHER ACTIVITIES**   SET / REPS / DISTANCE   TIME

....
....
....
....
....

NOTES

....
....

🕐 6A 7 8 9 10 11 12P 1 2 3 4 5 6 7 8 9 10+

B=BREAKFAST   L=LUNCH   D=DINNER   S=SNACKS   E=EXERCISE

DAY

MO TU WE TH FR SA SU

DATE ....

HOW I FEEL

BREAKFAST	LUNCH	DINNER
....	....	....
....	....	....
....	....	....
....	....	....
....	....	....
_____ ___		

SNACKS

....
....
....

TOTAL CALORIES

_____ ___

PROTEIN CONTENT   FIBER CONTENT

_____ _____

WEIGHT   SLEEP   WATER   PROTEIN

OTHER

....

♡ EXERCISE / OTHER ACTIVITIES   SET / REPS / DISTANCE   TIME

....	....	....
....	....	....
....	....	....
....	....	....
....	....	....

NOTES

....
....

🕐 6A 7 8 9 10 11 12P 1 2 3 4 5 6 7 8 9 10+

B=BREAKFAST   L=LUNCH   D=DINNER   S=SNACKS   E=EXERCISE

HOW I FEEL

:smiley: :smile: :neutral: :frown:
O O O O

MO TU WE TH FR SA SU

DATE ....

DAY (90)

BREAKFAST	LUNCH	DINNER

SNACKS

TOTAL CALORIES
_____

PROTEIN CONTENT FIBER CONTENT

WEIGHT   SLEEP   WATER   PROTEIN

OTHER ....

:heart: **EXERCISE / OTHER ACTIVITIES**   SET / REPS / DISTANCE   TIME

NOTES

....

....

:clock: 6A 7 8 9 10 11 12P 1 2 3 4 5 6 7 8 9 10+

B=BREAKFAST L=LUNCH D=DINNER S=SNACKS E=EXERCISE

DAY 90

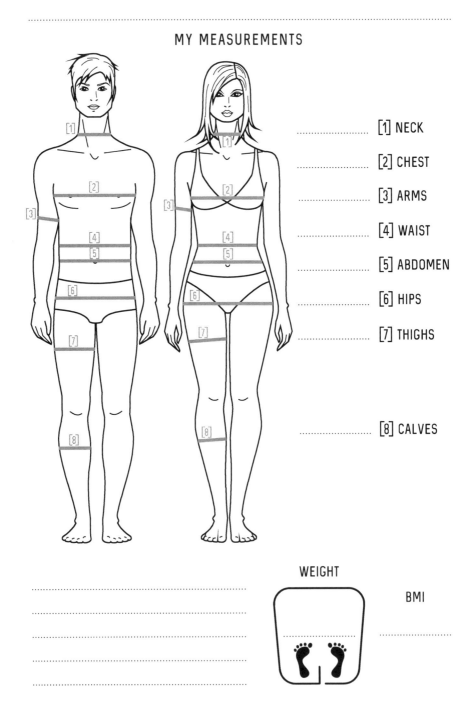

MY MEASUREMENTS

.... [1] NECK

.... [2] CHEST

.... [3] ARMS

.... [4] WAIST

.... [5] ABDOMEN

.... [6] HIPS

.... [7] THIGHS

.... [8] CALVES

WEIGHT

BMI

MY RESULTS

DAY 1	DAY 90		DIFFERENCE
....	....	[1] NECK	....
....	....	[2] CHEST	....
....	....	[3] ARMS	....
....	....	[4] WAIST	....
....	....	[5] ABDOMEN	....
....	....	[6] HIPS	....
....	....	[7] THIGHS	....
....	....	[8] CALVES	....

WEIGHT

WEIGHT

WEIGHT

BMI

BMI

BMI

NOTES